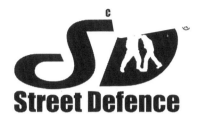

Street Defence

SELF DEFENCE FOR THE STREETS 'DEFENCE NOT ATTACK'

"The sole aim of the Street Defence system is to make people feel safe and to reduce fatalities or serious injuries to innocent/vulnerable individuals"

COLIN LEE BERRY

Please note that the publisher and author of this instructional book are NOT RESPONSIBLE in any manner whatsoever for any injury or litigation that may result from practising the techniques and/or following the instructions given within. Martial arts and self-defence training can be dangerous both to you and to others if not practiced safely. If you're in doubt as to how to proceed or whether your practice is safe, consult with a trained martial arts instructor/self-defence instructor before beginning. Since the physical activities described herein may be too strenuous in nature for some readers, it is also essential that a physician be consulted prior to training.

www.streetdefenceuk.com

CONTENTS

PREFACE   5

AUTHOR PROFILE   7

STREET DEFENCE TESTIMONIALS   9

INTRODUCTION 'DEFENCE NOT ATTACK'   11

GOOD PRACTICE AND COMMON SENSE   13

BEING PREPARED   16

THE REACTION GAP   19

THE STREET DEFENCE SYSTEM - ARMED   22

STANCES & FOOTWORK   24

MOVEMENT   27

MYTH OR FACT 1   28

STRIKES   29

MYTH OR FACT 2   37

CHOKE ESCAPE CONCEPTS   38

CLINCH CONTROL CONCEPTS   45

MYTH OR FACT 3   49

KNIFE DEFENCE CONCEPTS   50

MYTH OR FACT 4   64

GUN DEFENCE CONCEPTS   65

GROUND ATTACKS - 3 SECOND RULE   75

OTHER WEAPON DEFENCE   85

RESTRAINING CONCEPTS   88

PRESSURE & WEAK POINTS   93

For Ria & Jayden

XXXXXX

PREFACE

After many years of studying a variety of martial art and self defence systems, I began to wonder if I could develop a system which brought everything together, whilst keeping the techniques as simple and direct as possible. The idea behind this is to make a system that anyone can pick up easily whether they have had plenty of martial arts/self defence knowledge or not. I developed and started teaching the Street Defence system in 2009 and have been teaching an array of different groups since then – children in schools, mental health nurses, security teams, police officers etc. I believe that the more complicated a self defence technique, the less likely it will be effective if needed and also it will be harder to remember in the height of an attack.

Since 2009, I have been constantly evolving the Street Defence system and will continue to do this indefinitely as I believe that there is never a complete system. I also believe that self defence is an important life skill in this current volatile world and therefore needs to be accessible for everyone. Self Defence and martial arts can be seen as intimidating by someone that has never trained in a system before and also experienced this many years ago when I started up. Another core element to my Street Defence system is to create an atmosphere where anyone would want to come along whilst teaching the most effective self defence techniques possible.

Hopefully in many years to come when I retire and pass the baton on to my children to carry on teaching, I want to know that I have taught many people how to defend themselves and prevented innocent people from being harmed. If my system saves at least one life, I would see that as a success. Martial arts and self defence is something I absolutely love and feel that everyone should have the ability to learn and be part of an amazing world with amazing martial art concepts all over the world.

AUTHOR PROFILE

COLIN LEE BERRY

- Street Defence Chief Instructor & Founder

- Fight Choreographer/Screen Combatant

- Celebrity Personal Trainer

- www.streetdefenceuk.com

Colin has been a martial arts enthusiast from a young age and has studied a variety of martial arts over the years. He trained in Tae Kwon Do and competed at the British (Silver Medal) and World Championship and found that this competition helped in developing his awareness in combat and how to evade being struck whilst trying to strike the fighter. Colin feels that you have to know how it feels to be in a fight situation before you can understand what works in combat and what does not.

Soon after competing for Tae Kwon Do, Colin moved his attention to Commando Krav Maga and became an instructor in 2007. After 2 years of being an instructor, Colin felt he had learnt enough over the years of training and studying to create his own concept. In 2009, Street Defence was born. Since 2009, Street Defence has gone from strength to strength and has been studied by an array of people/groups. Colin adapts the system to suit the individual or group.

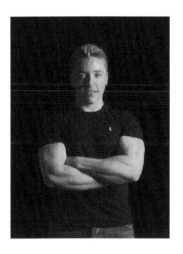

Colin has also been a personal trainer since 2001 and has integrated his knowledge into his classes as the fitter you are, the more likely you are to survive an attack. If you can't run away from a knife attack because you are out of condition, that could cost you your life.

STREET DEFENCE TESTIMONIALS

"Colin has worked at Haileybury for two years delivering a five week self-defence course for year 11 students. He has an excellent relationship with the pupils, balancing the informality of the nature of this type of session with the need for there to be order and clarity of purpose. The students enjoy the sessions and gain a great deal from them. Colin is reliable, punctual, and well organised. He comes highly recommended."

Ann Spavin - Teacher at Haileybury and Imperial Service College

"This system is easy to learn, practical in its application, builds confidence and I found it to be invaluable when faced with violent confrontations"

Paul Clarke – MET Police Sergeant

"A well put together system".

Peter Consterdine - Joint Director & Chief Instructor of The British Combat Association

"Colin's Street Defence service was absolutely ideal for what I was looking for. I hadn't taken any Martial Arts classes before and was looking for someone to teach me practical self-defence skills that would be easy to learn and effective. I was quickly impressed with Colin's unique system that combines the most practical elements of various Martial Arts forms, helping you to know how to defend yourself in any street situation. Training with Colin has been a really enjoyable experience - it has built my confidence and most importantly, has equipped me with invaluable skills in self-defence. I would highly recommend his services!"

Tania Diggory - Dance Instructor, Founder & Managing Director of United Grooves

INTRODUCTION 'DEFENCE NOT ATTACK'

The concept of the Street Defence system is that it is only used in defence not attack. If an attack is brought upon us or an attack is imminent then techniques are needed to neutralise the threat.

Street Defence has been developed so it can be learnt quickly and easily. The learner will be proficient in defending themselves from an array of attacks. This system has also been developed to mirror the attacks that commonly occur on the streets of many westernised societies.

Too many systems look at techniques that are too technical and would take many years to master. Many systems also use defence techniques against attacks that are unlikely to occur.

Although we are able to defend ourselves once skilled in the techniques of Street Defence, we must use sound judgement on how much force is used against an attacker. Our priority is to control the situation and remove the need to defend ourselves as acting calmly can reduce the threat of an attack from happening.

Legally the force used against an attacker can only reflect the force used against us. If we get out of a threatening situation but have used excessive force then we could face prosecution by the police. An example of this would be if an attacker pushes you up against the wall in a clinch, you then unlock the clinch followed up with an elbow strike to create distance between you and the attacker. This is a fine response although if we were to then carry on throwing punches and kicks especially if the attacker is on the floor, then this would be seen as excessive force. We had done enough by getting out of the clinch and creating distance. The only reason that we should have used anymore techniques is if the attacker comes in with further attacks.

The concept behind the system is not only to teach people techniques of how to defend themselves; it has been designed so that the defender reacts without thinking. If we have to think about how we are going to defend against an attack; it's too late. The only way to react without thinking is to have continual training in this system. Only with constant drills and training will the student be learning to react rather than think.

GOOD PRACTICE AND COMMON SENSE

After teaching self-defence for many years I have trained many students who have started at my classes after being threatened or at the receiving end of an attack or mugging. This information has allowed me to help many students be able to become more observant and avoid potentially violent situations.

NIGHTS OUT:

1. When on nights out with a group of friends, always remember to make sure everyone gets home safely at the end of the night. I have heard many times how someone has been attacked as all their friends disappeared and they had no other way of getting home other than walk miles in the dark. This immediately makes you a target to attackers. If you find yourself in this position get yourself to a public area as soon as possible then try to contact anyone to come and get you. Even borrow a phone to make a call if your phone battery has died.

2. Do not take too much money with you. If you are held up during or after a night out, this gives the muggers less to get away with. Take enough cash for what you need and a debit or credit card which you can easily cancel if need be. As for phones,

buy a cheap phone which you can use on nights out rather than an expensive smart phone which mugger's target.

3. **Pre arrange lifts home.** Rather than pick up a cab outside a venue, organise a lift home with a friend or family member (that has not been drinking themselves). Opportunists are known to pretend to be cab drivers and have a sinister agenda or are trying to make some money illegally and to top it off they probably won't have any car insurance in the event of an accident.

4. **Stay in groups.** Always stay in your circle of friends and never leave anyone behind or let them walk home on their own. You are less likely to be targeted if you are in a group.

5. **Always look after your drink.** Whilst in bars and clubs, never leave your drink unattended. If you have lost sight of your drink for a period of time, you will not be sure it hasn't been tampered with (drugs). If you do lose sight of your drink, go and buy another one.

6. **Stay in brightly lit/public areas.** If you find yourself on your own or you have decided against the advice above and walk home alone, always stick to brightly lit and public areas. Muggers/ attackers always want to target vulnerable people.

7. **Never flash the cash.** When paying for drinks or at cash points, never show off how much cash you have on you. I have worked with a couple

of people in the past that have been mugged because they were seen at the bar with hundreds of pounds in cash when paying for drinks. The attackers waited for this guy to leave the bar on his own and mugged him.

BEING PREPARED

Cheaper 2nd Phone: If you are travelling or on a night out there is no point in taking an expensive £400+ phone out with you. Simply buy a cheap 2nd phone which you can switch your sim over to. That way if it gets stolen, apart from the chip you won't be out of pocket anywhere near as much. Also by taking out a cheap phone, you instantly become less of a target from potential muggers.

Emergency Cash Keyring: Unfortunately if you do get mugged whilst travelling or on a night out you can be left with no money to get home etc. A couple of years ago I bought this cheap keyring which allows you to roll up a bank note inside. This inventive keyring will allow you to get home because if you have your money and phone taken you will have no other way of getting home.

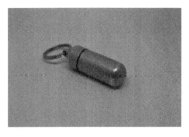 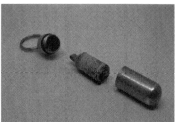

Metal Card Holder: Unfortunately criminals are getting more clever with regards to stealing people's money. Now that we can pay for items/services by just touching our bank/credit cards on a card terminal, some criminals have found a way of hiding one of these terminals in their jackets then walk along busy train carriages etc. and brush past people who have their cards in just their wallet or within their phone holder. £20-£30 does not sound like too much to lose individually, but imagine if they spend a few hours doing this. Therefore invest in a credit/debit card holder which is metal and prevents these criminals being able to scan your cards.

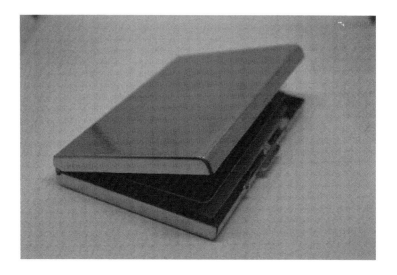

Golf Umbrella: Living in England can mean carrying an umbrella is a pretty standard thing to have. If you walk home late at night from work or through a dark and dingy underground car park to your car, a golf umbrella with the metal spike at the end can give you a barrier between you and a potential attacker. I have known a couple of people to use a golf umbrella to fend an attacker off so can come in useful.

Car Keys: Most of us carry a set of keys around with us all of the time. If you don't have many keys (1 or 2) on your key set then I would recommend you get a few more keys to add to the chain. The myth of carrying your keys between your fingers if you are walking down a dark alleyway on your own late at night is a good thing to do is not the best of ideas as you can cause a lot of damage to your own hand if you punched an attacker. I would recommend holding a couple of the keys in your hand and letting the other keys loose from your grip. If an attacker was to lunge toward you, you can flick/slash the loose keys towards their face and again like the golf umbrella, it acts as a barrier that the attacker needs to get through in order to cause you harm.

Distractions: The art of distraction can be invaluable when confronted by an attacker. If you are going to have to perform a strike in order to get away from a confrontation safely, just throwing an object like a hat or loose change towards the attackers face just before you

THE REACTION GAP

You should allow a 4-6 feet gap between you and the attacker (even though this is not always possible). This allows you to look into the person's eyes and can still see their feet. The advantages of this Reaction Gap are:

It will give you more time to react and respond to any aggression.

It means that you won't have to invade the person's personal space. This may help read anxiety and prevent them from becoming violent.

THE IMPORTANCE OF LEARNING AND PRACTISING YOUR DISTANCES FROM YOUR OPPONENT

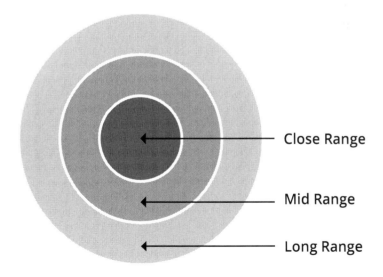

Close Range

Mid Range

Long Range

During your training sessions with other students, you must learn to detect what distance your attacker is at (close, mid or long range). Once you know what range the attack is coming from you will be able to use the appropriate techniques. This can vary from student to student because of lever length etc. The more skilful you become, the further away the threat will be as your awareness and observation has detected the threat way before the attacker has got close enough. The only threat that you want to be close to is the gun hold up situation. It is easier for you to get out of the line of fire if you are close to the gun rather than far away.

GREEN = LONG RANGE

Even though this threat gives you a lot more time to react than the red zone, the threat is still imminent. And like any of the zones on the diagram above, you need to react instantly.

AMBER = MID RANGE

When the threat reaches this zone, your reaction time is dramatically reduced to that of the red zone (long range). Your techniques will vary to those of the green zone and this range should mean you are able to reach out and make contact with the attacker's wrist or weapon. If this is not possible, the threat will still be in the green zone and must be dealt with accordingly.

RED = SHORT RANGE

This range includes if the weapon or threat is in a hold up or static scenario (knife to throat etc.). If the threat is static in a hold up this should make it easier to neutralise the threat or disarm the weapon as a static target is always easier to hit or control. If the threat is at short range and is a moving threat (knife thrust etc.), you must do whatever necessary to move your body away from the threat to enable you to compose yourself to deal with the threat or you must move in and take the opponent out.

THE STREET DEFENCE SYSTEM - ARMED

The Street Defence System has 5 levels of how the student conducts themselves in order to survive or prevent an attack.

AWARENESS

The main problem with most attacks that occur is that people are often not aware of their surroundings. If you can sense a threat before it even happens then not only would you be ready to defend yourself, you may also be able to avoid the situation by staying away from the threat or leaving the area. Most of the time the best action to take is to run and avoid the threat altogether. Even if you are highly skilled, things can go wrong and it is not worth risking your life.

RELAX

The most natural response to a threat is to become tense, nervous and/or aggressive. However the best response is to be calm and relaxed as possible. This may even calm the attacker down due to the fact that they see that you do not want to fight. It is also proven that if you are tense and then go to react, you can slow down your response. Although, if you relax and then react your whole body fires into action.

MANAGE

This is as the title describes. We control the situation, whether it is gaining a lock or control of the weapon.

ESTABLISH CONTROL

Once the attacker has been controlled we need to act so that the attack has been ended and there is no risk of a further attack from the attacker. This could be that you now have complete control of the weapon or you are in the position that the attacker is now grounded and is no longer a threat.

DEPART

Again as the title suggests, once the threat has been neutralised and there is no risk of a further threat, leave the scene and make your escape.

STANCES & FOOTWORK

Footwork is the base at which all your techniques are applied. If your footwork and stances are not up to standard then your techniques will falter.

STANCE

The correct Street Defence stance creates a firm base which gives stability, balance and a good position to apply your techniques and at the same time, keep yourself protected. If we are trying to prevent an attack, we should have our feet square to the attacker with our hands out in front of us. This gives the attacker the impression that we do not want to fight. Although if it is needed, we can move straight into a palm strike.

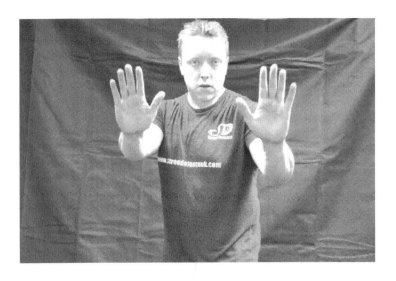

However if the threat of a lunging knife attack is imminent, we should adopt the following stance:

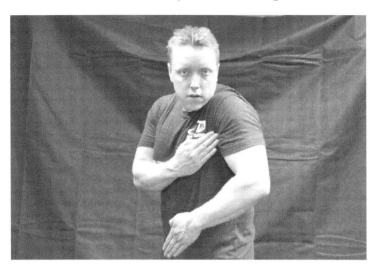

If a slashing knife attack is brought upon us, the following stance should be adopted:

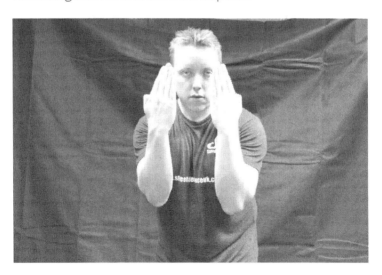

(Orthodox position) – adopt a stance with the left foot forward, thus delivering the most powerful technique with the right hand (Cross).

(Southpaw) – adopt a stance with the right foot forward. This allows them to drive off the back left foot and deliver a more powerful left handed strike.

HAND/ARM POSITIONING (BASED ON STANDING IN ORTHODOX POSITION)

Your left arm should be in front of you with your palm facing towards you and your forearm should be horizontal to the floor in a shield like position. Your rear arm should be across your body palm facing in, as if to protect your heart. Remember to tuck your chin in to your left shoulder to help defend against any throat attack.

The aim with the hand/arm positioning used with the Street Defence system is so to protect your body as much as possible and to also be in a position to easily perform a technique.

FOOT POSITION

The rear foot should be positioned at a 45 degree angle with the heel slightly raised off the ground. The weight should be slightly on the ball of the rear foot and the front foot flat. This allows you to shift forwards.

MOVEMENT

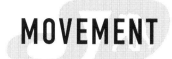

When moving it is important to remain in the stance as above unless you are trying to prevent an attack. This will maximise your balance, stability and safety.

Once you have mastered the basic moves of the Street Defence system, the heel raise and movement can be sped up by pushing off the balls of the feet in a shuffling action.

However the feet must never meet or cross when moving as this reduces your base of support. Therefore you lose balance and power and make yourself vulnerable to be taken to the ground.

• To move forward, lead with the front foot

• To move backwards, lead with the back foot

• To move left, lead with the left foot

• To move right, lead with the right foot

REMEMBER: A MOVING TARGET IS HARDER TO HIT

MYTH OR FACT 1

'If I have to strike an attacker I should punch him as hard as possible'

Answer = Myth:

If you can avoid confrontation at any point then do it. If you have no choice but to strike an attacker you should be looking at palm striking to the face rather than punching. Palm strikes massively reduce the chance of injury to your hand and wrist. Many boxers who have been involved in street fights have ended up breaking knuckles etc. proving that punching can cause damage yourself especially as these are people who know how to punch. In boxing and many martial arts, gloves are worn to spar and for bag work. You will not be wearing these if a surprise attack comes your way.

STRIKES

Although striking is a main ingredient in most martial art or self defence systems, most situations do not require you to make a strike. Striking is not always the best way to resolve a dispute or aggressive situation and if you do strike and it is not a relevant response to the threat then you could be prosecuted. However in some situations you have no choice. It can be a matter of hit or be hit. If you feel like your life and health is in danger from being struck by the aggressor then sometimes striking is the only option.

Like all the techniques in this book, striking needs to be constantly practised in order to perfect technique and to improve the speed when performing the strike. It does not matter how powerful your strikes are, if they are not performed quickly and efficiently, it could mean you get hit before you have been able to unleash your strike.

STRIKES:

- Palm Heel Strike – Cross

- Hammer Fist – Cross

- Elbow Strike - Right

- Rhino Strike/Punch Defence

- Groin Strike

PALM HEEL STRIKE (CROSS):

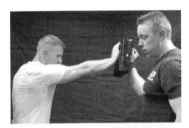 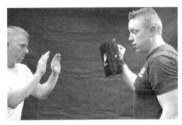

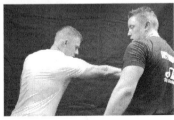

HAND POSITION:

The part of the hand that is used to strike the opponent is the bottom part of your palm with your fingers back (Fingers do not make contact).

MOVEMENT (STRIKING WITH RIGHT HAND):

Whilst in the orthodox stance and palms facing forward in a non-threatening manner, slightly lift your left foot off of the ground and drive forward using the right foot. As soon as the left foot has made contact with the ground, drive your right hand forward (with the bottom of your palm) whilst pushing the right hip through. You should feel the weight and momentum of your body through the sudden burst forward give you the power to make the strike count.

HAMMER FIST (CROSS):

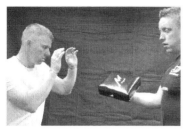 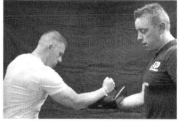

HAND POSITION:

Your fist should be clenched with the thumb over the top of the index fingers. You should strike with the bottom of the clenched fist in a downward fashion.

MOVEMENT (STRIKING WITH RIGHT HAND):

Whilst in the orthodox stance and palms facing forward in a non-threatening manner, slightly lift your left foot off of the ground and drive forward using the right foot. At the same time your right hand should be made into a clenched fist. As soon as the left foot has made contact with the ground, begin to rotate your body to the left with a slight lift then sudden drop of your body weight. You should use this to help give power to the downward strike of the hammer fist.

ELBOW STRIKES (RIGHT):

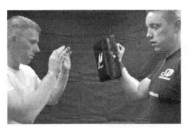 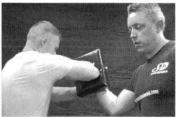

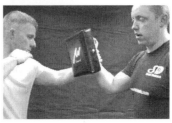

MOVEMENT:

Whilst in the orthodox stance and palms facing forward in a non-threatening manner, slightly bring your right hand across your body with your fist almost in contact with your chest. Explosively rotate to your left with your elbow pointing at your attacker. Aim a few inches to the left of the attacker's face. Therefore you will be hitting through the target and not at it.

RHINO DEFENCE/ATTACK

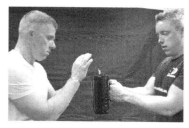 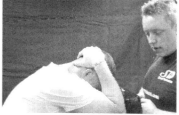

AIM: To defend against all punches aimed at your head (straight or hook punches) and at the same time using the blocking arms as an attack.

START POSITION:

Place your hands out In front of you with your palms facing towards your attacker (On Guard).

DISARM:

- As you feel that a punch technique is going to be used by your attacker, bring your hands around the back of your head with the palms in contact with your head.

- At the same time, have the elbows pointing forwards with your forearms in contact with your temples.

- This should act as a protection for all the vulnerable areas of your head.

- A split second after your hands and arms are in position, lift your front foot (left) slightly off of the ground and propel yourself forward as fast and as powerful as you can towards the attacker.

- Drive the point of your elbows into your attacker's mid-section.

- When the technique is used effectively any punch to your head should be blocked as well as making an impact to neutralise the threat of your attacker.

GROIN KICK (RIGHT):

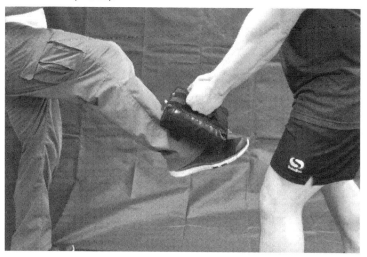

START POSITION:

Adopt the guard position.

MOVEMENT:

Look forward lifting the front knee to a 90 degree angle. Ensure that the foot of the back leg is turned out at a 45 degree angle. Extend the front leg (push don't flick out the leg) to 95% of its full reach aiming to strike with the ball of the foot and not the toes.

ENHANCING YOUR STRIKING TECHNIQUE:

When you strike, it is not just the arm and hand that the power generates from. Your whole body should work as one to create the power needed to strike with optimal power. The movement originates from the rear foot. The rear foot acts like a spring and allows you to propel your body forward and if you hit whilst driving forward with perfect technique, you will generate the power needed to perform the strike.

In order to improve your technique and power you definitely need to work with a training partner. Once you get into the perfect movement, you should then begin to test your distances from the attacker (strike pad). The further away you are from the attacker and are able to strike with full power the better. If you find that you have to almost be on top of the pad to perform the strike with power then you really need to practise moving further away.

MYTH OR FACT 2

'If an attacker is bigger or stronger than me, I have no chance of defending myself'

Answer = Myth:

This is a statement I hear many people say before they start training in the Street Defence system. As you will later see in the Pressure Point/Weakness Concepts section of this book, it does not matter how big or strong and attacker is, everyone's throat, eyes and groin are as weak as anyone's. As a last resort if this is all you have left to prevent serious harm being done to yourself, strike, grab, gouge or twist any of these areas and I am sure you will get the desired response which will create an opening for you to escape.

Also if you practise and study Street Defence consistently to perfect your skills, you will begin to unlock the true power that your body can generate. Once you see your power increase, your confidence will also rise. Confidence I believe is also another factor in making an attacker think twice about attacking you. Attackers tend to pick vulnerable and easy targets.

CHOKE ESCAPE CONCEPTS

With a full on choke, you have only 6-8 seconds of air before you pass out.

Chokes are performed around the throat area and are used to either a static or moving attack (pushing). Due to only 6-8 seconds left of air when a full on choke is performed, the need to escape as quickly as possible is essential. Whether it is a groin strike, eye gouge or rotation technique that causes pressure on the attacker's wrist to release the choke, the move has to be performed quickly. If you don't get out of the choke, you risk passing out, death or more attacks as you lay motionless on the floor.

Chokes can either occur when static (against a wall or where you are standing) or when the choke is being performed with the attacker pushing you back at the same time. With all the defensive moves in this area, you need to establish your balance as quickly as possible otherwise you are at an even higher risk of severe injury by now being on the floor.

The chokes covered in this area are:

- Front Choke Escape – Groin/Septum Strike
- Front Choke – Elbow drop/Strike
- Side Headlock
- Rear Headlock

FRONT CHOKE ESCAPE – GROIN/SEPTUM STRIKE

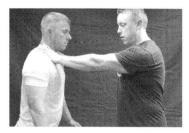 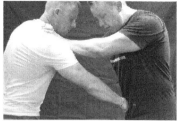

AIM: To release the choke before you lose consciousness.

START POSITION:

Restore balance before you are pushed to the ground and then to release the choke before you lose consciousness. Move your body into a quarter squat positions at a 45 degree angle to restore balance.

DISARM:

- Once balance has been restored, using the inner arm, strike the attacker with a back fist strike to the groin or stomach. Or an eye gouge can be performed with the same hand.

- After the groin or stomach strike, using a palm heel strike to the attacker's nose in a wave like motion, this will tip the attacker back and to the floor.

- Once this has been performed, make your escape and leave the scene.

FRONT CHOKE ESCAPE – ELBOW DROP/STRIKE

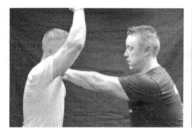 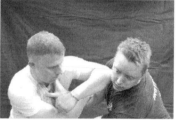

AIM: To release the choke before you lose consciousness.

START POSITION:

Restore balance before you are pushed to the ground and then to release the choke before you lose consciousness.

DISARM:

• Bring your left arm up and across the attacker's grip around your throat.

• Drop your body weight down onto the attacker's arm.

• The attacker will be slightly off balance.

• Then rotate your body to the right whilst striking the attacker across the face with your right elbow.

SIDE HEADLOCK ESCAPE

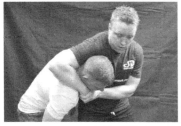
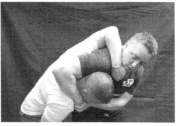
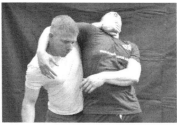

AIM: To release the headlock before you lose consciousness.

START POSITION:

(Headlock in the right arm of the attacker). As the headlock is in full force, pull your head away from the attacker. This prevents the attacker from easily pulling you to the floor.

DISARM:

- Lift your left arm up by the side of your body and place the blade of your hand underneath the attacker's nose.

- Put your left foot, heel positioning into the ground behind the attacker's feet.

- Apply pressure to the attacker's nose and flip the attacker over your left leg.

- Once the attacker is on the floor, leave and make your escape.

REAR HEADLOCK ESCAPE

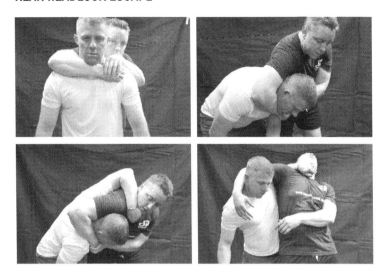

AIM: To release the headlock before we lose consciousness.

START POSITION:

(Headlock in the right arm of the attacker) As the headlock is in full force, get ready to drop your body weight to the right of the attacker.

DISARM:

- Drop your body weight and roll your body into position of the side headlock.

- Turn your head away from the attacker; this prevents the attacker from easily pulling you to the floor.

- Lift your left arm up by your side and place the blade of your hand underneath the attacker's nose.

- Put your left foot, heel positioning into the ground behind the attacker's feet.

- Apply pressure to the attacker's nose and flip the attacker over your left leg.

- Once the attacker is on the floor, leave and make your escape.

CLINCH CONTROL CONCEPTS

The only difference between clinch control and choke escapes is that you do not have the initial worry of the attacker trying to make you pass out or worse. However, with a choke, there are many other scenarios that can come from a clinch. A head butt is a common threat from a clinch a long with a punch if you are in a one handed clinch.

Like all the other techniques in this book, you need to release the clinch (threat) as soon as possible and neutralise the threat and escape as quickly as possible.

The clinch control techniques covered in this area are:

- Double Hand top grab – Elbow drop/Strike

- Single Hand top grab – Arm knock/Hammer Fist

- Rear Top Grab – Arm lock and strike

DOUBLE HAND TOP GRAB – ELBOW DROP/STRIKE

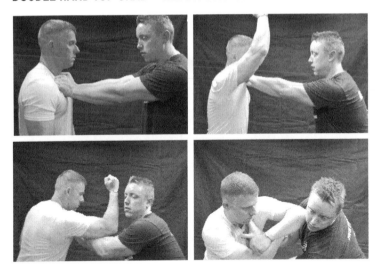

AIM: To neutralise the threat as soon as possible before it escalates.

START POSITION:

Drop your right foot back to restore balance.

DISARM:

- Bring your left arm up and across the attackers grip around your throat.

- Drop your body weight down onto the attackers arm.

- The attacker will be slightly off balance.

- Then rotate your body to the right whilst striking the attacker across the face with your right elbow.

SINGLE HAND TOP GRAB

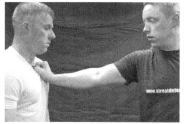 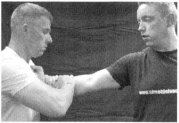

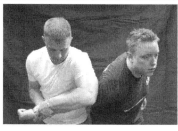

AIM: To neutralise the threat as soon as possible before it escalates.

START POSITION:

Slightly drop your body weight to maintain balance.

DISARM:

- Whilst rotating your body to your right, knock the attacker's left arm with your right forearm with your elbow higher than your wrist.

- Rotate hard to knock the attacker's left hand grip away from you.

- As soon as the left hand grip is gone, use the same hand and quickly rotate back left with a hammer fist strike to the attacker's face using your right hand.

- Follow this strike up with a left palm heel strike.

REAR CHOKE – ARM LOCK/STRIKE

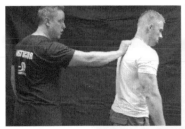 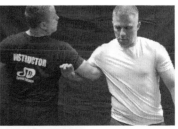

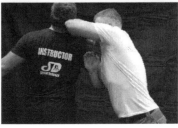

AIM: To release the grab before you get pulled backwards to the ground.

START POSITION:

Place the left foot forward to restore some form of balance.

DISARM:

- Once you have restored balance, lift your right arm up and begin to rotate your body to your right.

- When you have turned to the point you are facing your attacker, hook your right arm all the way round the attacker's arms and lock them in place.

- As the lock is activated then strike with a palm heel or elbow strike with your left arm.

MYTH OR FACT 3

'I should run if I see someone approaching with a knife'

Answer = Fact:

Even if you feel you have the ability and the confidence to defend yourself and use techniques against a knife attack, I do not see the point in taking the risk if you are able to run and avoid the situation altogether. However if you do not feel you are able to outrun the attacker and have no choice but to defend against a knife attack then you have no choice but to face it.

KNIFE DEFENCE CONCEPTS

One of the most violent crimes that occur on the streets of today is knife attacks. Unfortunately this means that learning to defend ourselves against a knife has never been so important. Studies have shown that due to the ease at which a knife or sharp object can be obtained by an attacker, this is the reason to why knife crime is so high.

As with gun disarming techniques, knife defence also has 3 ranges of defence. The threat can be close (touching), mid-range or long range (arm's length or lunging attack).

Knife attacks tend to be performed from various angles which are why the knife, at close range can be seen to be more threatening than a gun at close range. This is due to the fact that once you are out of the line of fire of a gun; you cannot be harmed by the gun. Also you do not have to be skilled to be deadly with a knife. Whereas a gun requires a bit more skill to operate to load, maintain and fire.

KNIFE DEFENCE:

Hold-Up (Close):

- Side of Throat (+Hand Grip)

- Across the Throat (+Hand Grip)

- Stomach (+Hand Grip)

Mid-Range Hold-up:

- Distraction + Strike

Mid-Range/Long Range Lunging Defence:

- Front deflection + Movement

- Front deflection + Strike

Slashing Defence:

- Knee Strike Counter (In Swinging)

- Arm Control (Out Swinging)

CLOSE RANGE: SIDE OF THROAT (KNEE STRIKE)

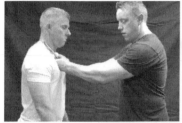 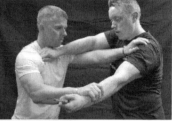

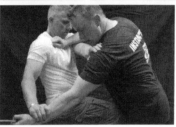

START POSITION:

Once the knife is placed to the side of your throat, your hands should be relaxed but held near to the threat of the knife. You should appear submissive so as to not intimidate the attacker in anyway.

DISARM (KNIFE IN ATTACKER'S RIGHT HAND):

- With your left hand slightly inside the knife wielding hand, push/deflect the hand to the right away from your throat and grab the wrist. Attempt to get your left arm as straight as you can.

- Then place your right hand on the attacker's right shoulder with your fingers partly down the back.

- Pull the attacker towards you with your right hand and drive your right knee into the attacker's groin. The knee strike should be repeated until the attacker is no longer a threat.

CLOSE RANGE: KNIFE ACROSS THE THROAT

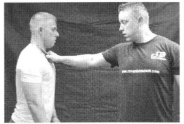
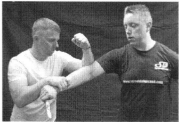

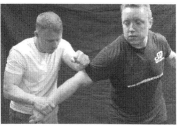

START POSITION:

Once the knife is placed across your throat, place your hands in a neutral/non-threatening position either side of the knife holding hand.

DISARM (KNIFE IN ATTACKER'S RIGHT HAND):

- Bring your right hand across your body and push the knife away from your throat and at the same time grab the wrist.

- Start to pull the attacker forward slightly and step in with your left foot.

- Place the bony part of your forearm slightly above the attacker's elbow of the knife holding arm. Start to rotate your body by stepping around with your right foot so you are almost facing the opposite direction to where you started.

- Place more pressure with your forearm whilst rotating even further. Whilst keeping hold of the attacker's wrist.

- Keep circling until the attacker is on the ground. The faster you perform this move, the more damage you will do to the attacker.

- When the attacker is on the floor, drop your nearside knee onto the back of the attacker's shoulder. Lift the knife holding arm up until the attacker drops the knife.

CLOSE RANGE: STOMACH

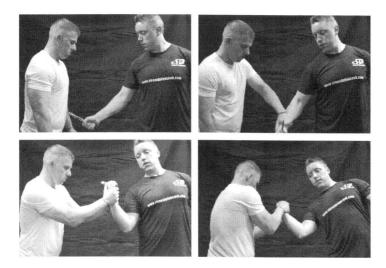

START POSITION:

Once the knife is placed around the stomach with the attacker in front of you, your hands should be relaxed and you should appear in a submissive position so as to not intimidate the attacker in anyway.

DISARM (DISARMING TO THE RIGHT):

- Cross the hands over the top of the attacking hand in a cross over position.

- Open the hands across so the attacking hand is re directed so the attacker's torso is exposed.

- Locking the attacking hand with the left hand, place the right hand on the attacker's right shoulder.

- Counter the move with a knee strike to the attacker's groin or mid-section.

MID-RANGE: DISTRACTION + STRIKE

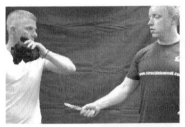 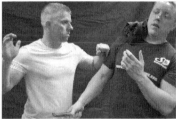

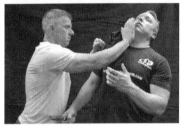

START POSITION:

This technique is used if you have something in your hand or are able to obtain an object that can be used as a distraction – money, phone etc.

DISARM (KNIFE IS IN THE ATTACKER'S RIGHT HAND):

- Try and relax and in no way signal that you are about to make a counter move, or this could result in the knife being thrust before the counter can be made.

- Throw the loose change, hat etc. at the attacker.

- This will create an opening for you to step in.

- With your hands out relatively wide, rotate your body to the right and at the same time you should strike the attacker's right hand with your left hand. Strike the hand so it moves across the attacker's body line.

- As the knife moves out of your knife line, drive your body forward and strike the attacker with your right hand – hammer fist or palm strike.

- Once the threat has been neutralised, leave the scene as quickly as possible.

MID/LONG RANGE: LUNGING DEFLECTION

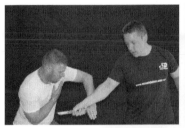 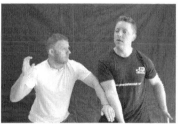

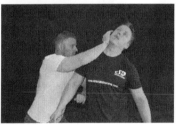

START POSITION:

As you perceive the lunging attack, place your left arm across the mid line of your body with your palm facing in. Have your right arm across your body covering your heart region.

DISARM (KNIFE IN THE ATTACKER'S RIGHT HAND):

- As the attack is coming in, open your defence (arms). Lifting your left elbow up and pointing forward with your hand pointing downwards and palm facing inwards. Your right arm should still be protecting your body (heart region). And tuck your chin into your left shoulder.

- As the attack is directed at you, deflect the wrist or lower forearm of the knife wielding arm to the right whilst also rotating your body to the right and moving your body to the left side of the attacker.

- Once you are at the left side of the attacker and have successfully deflected the knife away, open your arm position and strike the attacker with a palm strike or a hammer fist strike.

- Once you have seen the attacker fall to the floor, leave the scene as quickly as possible.

MID RANGE: SLASHING – TAKE DOWN (INSWINGING)

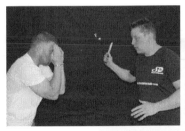 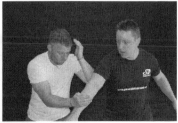

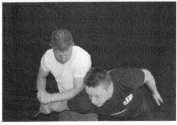

START POSITION:

Have both of your arms protecting your body with your forearms parallel, with your palms facing each towards you.

DISARM (KNIFE IN THE ATTACKER'S RIGHT HAND):

- Lean your body back as the knife moves across your body line.

- As the knife passes, spring off the rear foot and step in towards the attacker's body.

- Block the attacker's arm with your arms in the same defensive position that you started in as the slashing arm is coming back across.

- Grab the knife wielding wrist with your right hand adding pressure with your left forearm in the attacker's shoulder.

- Lift the attackers wrist higher that the level of the shoulder. Add more pressure until the attacker is free of the knife.

MID RANGE: SLASHING – KNEE STRIKE (OUTSWINGING)

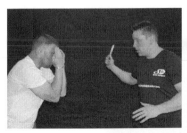 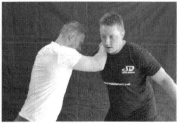

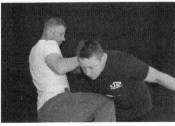

START POSITION:

Have both of your arms protecting your body with your forearms parallel, with your palms facing each towards you.

DISARM (KNIFE IN THE ATTACKER'S RIGHT HAND):

- As the knife is outwards of the attacker's body line, step in towards the attacker.

- As the knife holding arm is on its way back towards you, make sure you are in close to the attacker and grab the arm with your left hand.

- Place your right hand on the attacker's right shoulder with your fingers gripped slightly over the back of the attacker's shoulder.

- Proceed to drive knee strikes into the attackers groin until the knife and/or the attacker fall to the floor.

ENHANCING YOUR KNIFE DEFENCE SKILLS:

Like most of the other areas of this book, you will need to train with a partner. Always start slowly with all training techniques in order to get comfortable using the technique. Once you can perform the technique well then ask your training partner to gradually build up the speed of the movement until you get to full speed.

If you are practising the hold-up knife defence techniques, then practise the techniques with your eyes shut or wearing a blindfold. If you can perform the techniques in these conditions then your confidence will massively improve as you are making the situation harder to perform by not using your sight.

When practising movement techniques – lunging attacks etc. start with your partner just holding the knife out in front so you can practise the technique. Like the hold-up training above, as you get more confident ask your training partner to slowly build the speed up of the knife as and when you are ready until you are at full speed. Also make sure your training partner is aiming for your mid-section. You want to know that you can perform the technique well. If they do not aim for you, you won't know if you are proficient at performing the technique or not.

MYTH OR FACT 4

'If I am confronted with a gun I should use a disarm technique as soon as possible'

Answer = Myth:

Even if you think you have the ability to successfully disarm the gun from the attacker, there is a risk. If you feel that the attacker just wants your money or phone etc. and that they will move on after, this may be the best option to take. We have to remember the main element of self-defence apart from avoiding confrontation where possible, is to escape from the situation unharmed. If the attacker points a gun at you requesting your money and phone, and you do as he says, he takes your belongings and runs off and you are unharmed then from a self-defence point of view this has been a success. On the flip side he might not just want to take your belongings, he may take this further and bring serious harm to you. With all threats, you have to make the judgement on whether you can run or perform the technique for the threat or hand over your belongings without getting harmed. The more you practice, the more you will know your ability and what is the best response for you to use.

GUN DEFENCE CONCEPTS

Even though gun crime is not at the same level as knife crime, guns are still a threat. Therefore techniques are required to enable us to get away from a vast array of attacks. Whether it is a threat from close, mid or long range (arm's length).

As well as learning techniques to physically disarm the gun from the attacker, you can also use verbal tactics. If the attacker wanted to shoot you, he would have done it already, therefore he wants something. It will tend to be your money, information or mobile phone that the attacker wants.

The main thing to do is to follow the attacker's commands. During your reply to the attacker you can perform the disarm technique. This will catch them out as they are waiting for the full response. Or you can come back with a random response that has nothing to do with the situation e.g. "Give me your money" (attacker), "Do you take MasterCard or Visa?"(Victim). This is then the technique will be performed as the attacker is trying to work out what you have just said. As you can see, if you are proficient in your techniques and you also use your verbal skills, you are more likely to be successful in disarming the gun from the attacker.

However if the gun is far out of reach from any techniques then you have to follow the orders of the attacker and hope that they close the gap.

GUN DEFENCE:

Hold-up (Close):

- Front Gun Disarm – Stomach/Chest

- Front Gun Disarm – Head

- Lower Back Gun Disarm – Same side

- Lower Back Gun Disarm – Opposite side/Knee Strike

- Lower Back Gun Disarm – Double Hand

CLOSE RANGE: FRONT GUN DISARM WITH ELBOW STRIKE (STOMACH/CHEST/HEAD)

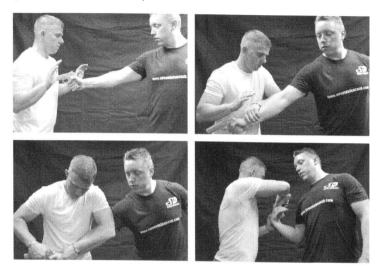

AIM: To disarm the weapon and gain our distance as soon as possible.

START POSITION:

Once the gun is placed at the stomach, chest or head area, your hands should be placed level with the gun. The hands should be relaxed and you should appear in a submissive position so as to not intimidate the attacker in any way.

DISARM (BASED ON TAKING THE GUN TO THE RIGHT OF YOUR BODY)

- Grabbing the wrist that is holding the gun with your left hand, rotate on the ball of your left foot.

- Pull the wrist round to the right side of your body, pulling the attacker slightly off balance and keeping the attackers wrist that is holding the gun in contact with your body.

- Place your right hand on top of the gun with your thumb underneath the hammer of the gun (preventing the gun from firing)

- Then rotate your body to your left with the attacker's wrist still in contact with your body and your right hand still clamped on top of the gun and aiming your right elbow at the attackers face.

- Follow through by pivoting on your right foot as you are rotating your body to the left.

- Once you have struck your attacker with your right elbow and disarmed the gun, gain your distance ASAP.

- Once you have gained your distance, demand the attacker to get to the floor in an authoritative fashion.

CLOSE RANGE: FRONT GUN DISARM TO HEAD (2)

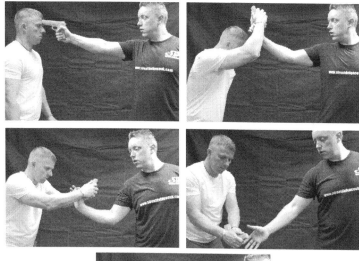

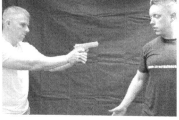

AIM: To disarm the weapon and gain our distance as soon as possible.

START POSITION:

- Once the gun is placed at your head, place your hands underneath the gun with your thumbs on the barrel of the gun with your thumbs side to side.

- At the same time you should quarter squat to take you out of the line of fire of the gun.

- Then you should push your thumbs towards the attacker whilst grabbing the gun.

- At the same time you should also step back with one foot which will help twist the gun out of the attacker's hands. You may also be lucky enough to be able to strike the opponent with the butt of the gun. Once you have obtained the gun from the attacker, point the gun back at the attacker and gain your distance ASAP.

CLOSE RANGE: BACK (REAR) GUN DISARM (LOW BACK, MID BACK) — SAME SIDE

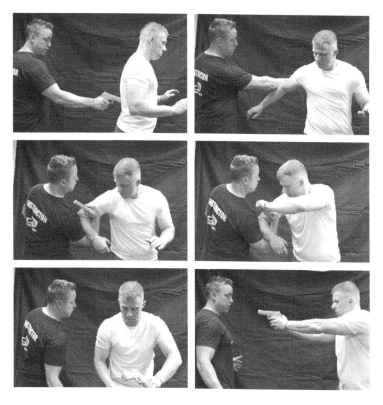

AIM: To disarm the weapon and gain your distance as soon as possible.

START POSITION:

Once the gun is placed at your lower back, your hands should be placed level with the gun. The hands should be relaxed and you should appear in a submissive position so as to not intimidate the attacker in anyway.

DISARM (DISARMING TO THE RIGHT):

- Deflect the gun with the back of your right hand whilst rotating your body to the right.

- Loop your right hand underneath the gun holding arm.

- Clamp the gun holding arm with your right arm and strike the attacker with your left elbow until the gun has dropped to the floor.

- Push the attacker away whilst your foot is on top of the gun.

- Then as before, demand the attacker to drop to the floor, if they haven't already whilst holding the gun.

CLOSE RANGE: BACK (REAR) GUN DISARM (LOW BACK, MID BACK) – OPPOSITE SIDE

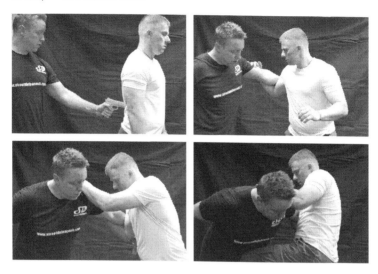

AIM: To disarm the weapon and gain your distance as soon as possible.

START POSITION:

Once the gun is placed at your lower back, your hands should be placed level with the gun. The hands should be relaxed and you should appear in a submissive position so as to not intimidate the attacker in anyway.

DISARM (DISARMING TO THE LEFT):

- Deflect the gun holding arm with your left forearm as you rotate. This will get you out of the line of fire.

- Step in towards the attacker and put your arms around the attacker thus clamping the gun holding arm against the attacker's body.

- Whilst holding the attacker as tight as possible, use your knee to strike the attacker's groin as many times as is needed.

- Do not let go of the attacker until the threat has been neutralised.

ENHANCING YOUR GUN DEFENCE SKILLS:

When practising with a partner, to improve your reactions, point the rubber gun at your training partner in any of the positions learnt so far. As soon as they disarm, they should point the gun straight back. In time, build up the speed of pointing the gun back and also vary the position you point the rubber gun as much as possible.

Like the knife, also try performing these techniques with your eyes shut or with a blindfold.

GROUND ATTACKS – 3 SECOND RULE

I f you find yourself on the floor, you have to be on your feet in no more than 3 seconds. This is due to other attackers joining in on the attack. Even though ground attacks are a major part of this course, we must realise that if we are proficient in our observation on the streets of today, we should never find ourselves in a position that we are on the floor with the attacker on top of us (either choking or punching etc.). However as this could still be a possibility, this section is still required in the event that it does happen.

In training, the 3 second rule is applied. This is due to the fact that we have to take into account that the attacker might have friends that will join in the attack if we are not back on our feet. 3 seconds is the standard time set and with training, it is easily executable.

Even though it should only take us 3 seconds to get out of the hold and back onto our feet, there are quite a few techniques rolled into one movement that need to performed at the same time for the move to be effective. However as with many techniques, if all else fails and the attack is seen to be life threatening or close enough, eye gouge techniques can be applied.

The idea behind this training is to show participants how to move when they are on the ground and to strike with their feet onto a strike shield that their partner is holding. The pad holder will also move around the person on the floor which will make them manoeuvre and keep the pad holder where their feet are for protection.

The techniques covered in this section are:

GROUND ATTACKS – 3 SECOND RULE

- Mounted Techniques – Between legs

- Mounted Techniques – Waistline

- Side Headlock on Floor

GROUND TO STAND

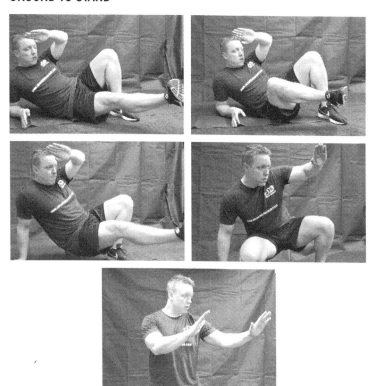

AIM: To protect yourself if you find yourself on the floor from kicks and/or punches and then to create an opening to which you can get to your feet and escape.

START POSITION

Turn your body onto the side (right). Steady yourself with your right arm. Your left arm is used as a last resort block to any attack coming towards your head. Your left foot/leg is used to guard and kick out at the attacker's shins or knees.

ESCAPE

Using your left leg to kick out at the attacker's shins and knees, as soon as you successfully strike the attacker and forces them backwards or to the ground, you need to get to your feet as soon as possible. To stand up quickly bring your left foot to the ground and use your right hand to raise your body off the ground. Then sweep your right foot back under your body and use it to bring you to a standing position. Always keep your guard throughout this movement. Once you are on your feet, escape immediately.

MOUNTED TECHNIQUES – BETWEEN LEGS

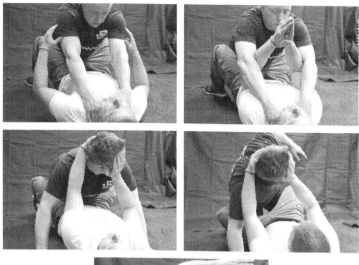

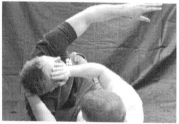

AIM: To release from the attack and get to the floor then away from the threat as soon as possible.

START POSITION:

To release from the choke, place both hands together in a praying position (palms together). Bring your hands up in between the choking hands until your hands are above your head. This will release you from the choke.

DISARM:

- To get the attacker off you, place your right hand flat on the attacker's left side of the face. Make sure that the edge of your right hand is alongside that of the attacker's nose.

- Place your left hand around the back of the attacker's head.

- Twist the attacker's head to the left, at the same time as lifting your right leg into the air.

- Whilst twisting the attacker's head to the left, place some pressure on the attacker's rib cage with your right leg. This will assist in rolling the attacker to the left of you.

- Keep twisting until you are now on top of the attacker. You should now have your right foot flat on the floor and be on your knee of your left leg with the attackers head in your hands.

- Strike the attacker's head on the ground and get to your feet as soon as you can, then leave the scene and the attacker.

MOUNTED TECHNIQUES – WAISTLINE

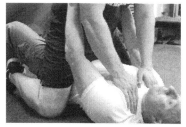 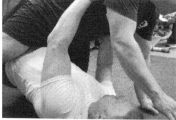

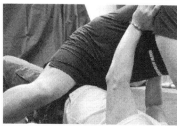

AIM: To release from the attack and get to the floor then away from the threat as soon as possible.

START POSITION:

To release from the choke, place both hands together in a praying position (palms together). Bring your hands up in between the choking hands until your hands are above your head. This will release you from the choke.

DISARM:

- Place your hands underneath the attacker's armpits.

- By activating your glute muscles (backside), lift your hips off the ground. But make sure you perform this at an angle as to lift the attacker over your right shoulder.

- At the same time as lifting the attacker up with your gluten muscles, use your hands to lift the attacker and throw them over your right shoulder.

- Once the attacker has been thrown, get to your feet as soon as you can and leave the scene.

DOUBLE KICK OUT

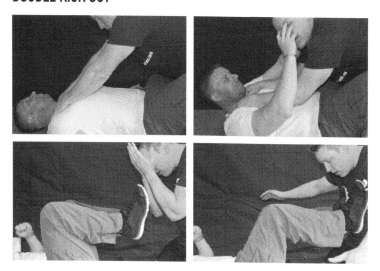

AIM: To release from the attack and get to the floor then away from the threat as soon as possible.

START POSITION:

To release from the choke, place both hands together in a praying position (palms together). Bring your hands up in between the choking hands until your hands are above your head. This will release you from the choke.

DISARM:

- To get the attacker off you. Place your fingers in an open position and place them in the attacker's eyes. This will force the attacker to move back to an almost sitting position.

- This will allow you to bring your knees and feet up towards yourself.

- Bring your feet up towards yourself, to the point that your backside is slightly off the ground.

- Then fire your feet towards the attacker's upper body (face or chest) with the heels of your feet.

- Get to your feet as soon as you can, then leave the scene and the attacker.

ENHANCING YOUR GROUND DEFENCE SKILLS:

When you are at a level where you feel comfortable with defending yourself on the ground in a training situation, start to bring in the 3 second rule. When training with your training partner, make sure they act as an attacker would by not allowing you to get out of the hold. An attacker in real life is not going to let you get out of the hold easily. Therefore you need to train in the same way. Once you can get off the floor in training within the 3 second time frame with your training partner resisting you, then you can feel more confident about getting out of a real life ground hold if the attack was to ever happen to you.

OTHER WEAPON DEFENCE

BASEBALL BAT DEFENCE – SPINNING DISARM (ORTHODOX POSITION)

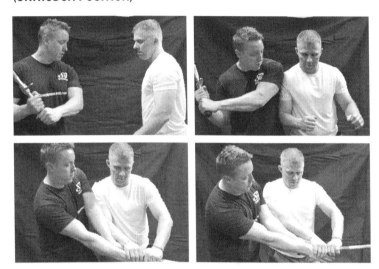

START POSITION:

Place your hands in front of your body with your palms facing towards the attacker at about shoulder level to the attacker. The idea is for this stance position to show that we do not want to fight and it also enables us to perform this technique a lot easier.

DISARM (BAT HELD IN THE ATTACKER'S RIGHT HAND SIDE):

- As the bat prepared for the swing (slightly moves backwards over the attackers shoulder), step in towards the attacker.

- Aim to get your right shoulder next to the left shoulder of the attacker and be as parallel to the attacker's body as possible.

- Place your hands near the forearms of the attacker.

- As the bat is in full swing, carry on rotating your body and slide your hands up the attackers arms until they are in contact and are gripping the bat.

- NEVER GRAB THE BAT!

- Once the attacker has swung through and you have control of the bat, the attacker will fall to the floor and you will have control of the bat.

- Then leave the scene as quickly as possible.

BOTTLE/OVER HEAD BAT DEFENCE

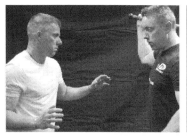
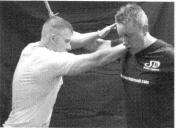

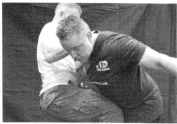

START POSITION:

Stand with your feet square on to the attacker with your hands out in front of you.

DISARM (BOTTLE OR BAT IS HELD IN THE ATTACKER'S RIGHT HAND):

- As the bottle or bat is brought back behind them to generate power for a strike, stand inside the path of the line of the weapon.

- Place your left arm straight above your head and step in towards the attacker.

- The bottle or bat arm will run down the side of left of your body.

- Then lock the right arm with your left arm then proceed to either elbow strike, palm strike or knee strike with your right side.

RESTRAINING CONCEPTS

For a complete self defence system, restraining has to form a major part of the syllabus. Ideally we want to prevent or leave before a situation escalates. However this is not always possible. The next level of response without having to strike and cause direct harm to the attacker, is to use a restraining technique in order to control an attacker which prevents them causing you or others harm. The idea would then be for others to help de-escalate the situation – a member of the public, police or security.

Over the years I have found a lot of martial art/self defence systems always look to strike. But restraining someone can not only help you or others being harmed but it can give the attacker time to calm down and prevent them from assaulting someone. In a strange way it could do the attacker a favour from getting arrested for assault.

However to perform restraining techniques just as any of the other techniques in this book, you need to know that you are proficient enough to perform the techniques effectively. If you are not, you could be putting yourself in the firing line by performing the technique badly which could lead to you getting seriously hurt.

THE TECHNIQUES COVERED IN THIS SECTION ARE:

- Arm Bar

- Rear Headlock Control

ARM BAR

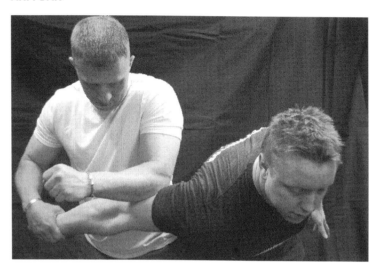

START POSITION:

With the attacker in front of you with their back to you. It is not always possible but if you can avoid the attacker knowing your position, that will give you even more time needed to perform the technique effectively.

DISARM:

- Approach the attacker from behind in a stealth like fashion.

- Grab the attacker's right wrist with your right hand and pull them slightly to the right and back towards you.

- Use the boney part of you left forearm and press this onto the attacker's right arm just above their right elbow where you will find a painful pressure point.

- Whilst adding pressure and turning you and the attacker to the right in a circular motion, begin to turn around clockwise as if you are going to guide them to the floor.

- You can hold the attacker in this position in a standing position. Just make sure that the attacker's right shoulder is lower than their right wrist.

- If you decide to take the attacker to the floor, continue with the circular downward spiral until the attacker ends up on the floor. Keep your body close if not touching the attacker on the way down so you end up dropping your weight on top of them instead of you hitting the floor. This may become painful for the attacker because they go to the floor but sometimes this may be your only option to control the attacker and prevent them causing you or others harm. The only problem with going to the floor is that it leaves you vulnerable to an attack from others (friends of the attackers). If this does happen, as you hit the floor the impact should at least stun the attacker and give you the time to spring up off the floor and escape as quickly as possible.

REAR HEADLOCK CONTROL

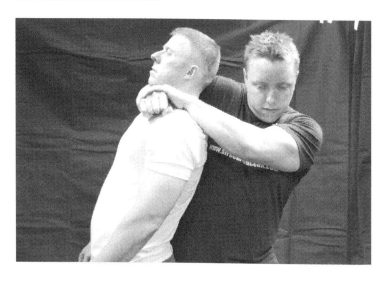

START POSITION:

Ideally you never want to have to restrain an attacker around the neck as this can be very dangerous. This technique should only be used in a violent/ life threatening scenario which may even involve the attacker holding a knife. Unlike the Arm Bar technique you have just learnt, the Rear Headlock Control technique can cause damage to the attacker. Therefore this technique should only be used if the threat requires it. Just like the Arm Bar you should position yourself behind the attacker ideally without them knowing of your whereabouts.

DISARM:

- If the attacker is taller than you, you will need to put a light stamp behind their right knee with your right foot, this will bring the attacker down to a lower level to make it easier to perform this restraining technique.

- Once the attacker has been brought to a more suitable level, place your right arm around their throat with your forearm central at the front of their neck.

- Whilst grabbing your right wrist with your left hand to seal the lock, drive your right hip into the lower back of the attacker to place them off balance towards you. You can hold them in this position until help arrives if needs be. However remember not to grab too tightly to the point the attacker passes out. If you start to feel the attacker becomes floppy then start to ease the lock around the neck of the attacker.

- Another option would be to throw the attacker to the floor. Rotate your body to your left, stepping slightly back with your left foot. As you twist to your left with speed, open the lock so the attacker is thrown to the floor to your left. This will allow you to escape as soon as possible.

PRESSURE & WEAK POINTS

The human body has so many pressure or weak points that pain can be inflicted without needing to punch or kick. When attacking weak points of the body, it should be seen as a last resort to ending an attack as the damage you can give the attacker is extremely high.

You are looking at life or death situations which would require maximal force in order to save you or someone else's life.

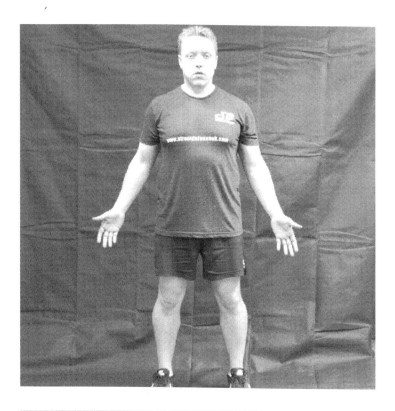

THE WEAK POINTS AND PRESSURE POINTS ON THE BODY ARE:

- Feet – foot stamps

- Shins – shin kicks

- Knees – knee stamp

- Groin

- Stomach

- Floating ribs

- Collar bone

- Throat

- Eyes

- Nose

- Ears